Best Practices in Teaching and Learning in Nursing Education

Linda Felver, PhD, RN
Barbara Gaines, EdD, RN
Marsha Heims, EdD, RN
Kathie Lasater, EdD, RN, ANEF
Gary Laustsen, PhD, APRN
Maggie Lynch, EdD
Launa Rae Mathews, MS, RN, COHN-S
Deb Messecar, PhD, MPH, RN
Joanne Noone, PhD, RN, CNE
Margaret Rhoads Scharf, DNP, PMHNP, FNP
Christine Tanner, PhD, RN, FAAN

National League
for Nursing

National League for Nursing
61 Broadway
New York, NY 10006
212-363-5555 or 800-669-1656
www.nln.org

ISBN 978-1-934758-13-7

Art Director, Mara Jerman

Printed in the United States of America

Best Practices in Teaching and Learning in Nursing Education

National League
for Nursing

Table of Contents

Dedication

We dedicate this monograph to the memory of our esteemed colleague, Dr. Marsha Heims, who passed away in June of 2010.

Dr. Heims, was an innovative, passionate, and extraordinary nurse educator. She was always in pursuit of the best available evidence for teaching and learning, never willing to settle for anything less than outstanding, and never shy about expressing her well-grounded point of view.

Introduction

Recent attention to pedagogy within higher education–and nursing education specifically–has focused on the paradigm shift toward learner-centered teaching (Barr & Tagg, 1995) and the need for new models of clinical education (Gubrud-Howe & Schoessler, 2008). Nursing educators everywhere face new challenges as technology expands our imaginations and the possibilities for teaching and learning.

This monograph presents evidence demonstrating how people learn and suggests best practices in teaching and learning with implications for curricular development. With the intention of guiding and motivating faculty towards implementation of the methods discussed, this document provides a platform for faculty development and a guide for administrators who must prioritize budget decisions. The considerations presented herein, supported by the literature, will serve as a framework for nursing faculty and administrators in the development of teaching and learning resources.

Overview and Guiding Principles for Identifying Best Practices

The discussion is divided into five sections, moving from broad evidence to specific suggestions:

- Research on Learning
- Evidence on Best Practices in Teaching and Learning in Higher Education
- Evidence on Aspects of Teaching and Learning in Nursing Education
- Evidence Regarding Pedagogical Strategies
- Faculty Development and Evaluation

Based upon the findings of the experts and researchers cited in literature on learning, several guiding principles are relevant to teaching and learning, and to the teaching and learning of nursing. These serve as the guiding principles upon which this document is based:

Learning is more effective when faculty use and reflect on best practices of teaching.

Learning is more effective when faculty decision-making is grounded in knowledge of best practices, student development, and nursing curricula.

Teaching and learning are more effective when appropriate resources are allocated to the teaching mission and when the teaching mission has administrative support.

Research on Learning

Bransford, Brown, and Cocking (2004) presented key findings about how people learn:

1. Students come to the classroom with preconceptions about how the world works. If their initial understanding is not engaged, they may fail to grasp the new concepts and information that are taught, or they may learn them for purposes of a test but revert to their preconceptions outside the classroom. (Students construct their learning based on what they know).

2. To develop competence in an area of inquiry, students must: (a) have a deep foundation of factual knowledge, (b) understand facts and ideas in the context of a conceptual framework, and (c) organize knowledge in ways that facilitate retrieval and application. (Students need a deep knowledge base and conceptual frameworks).

3. A "metacognitive" approach to instruction which defines learning goals can help students take control of their learning and monitor their progress in achieving learning goals (see Appendix for a glossary of terms, including metacognition).

Weimer (2002) focused on the change in emphasis and attention from teaching to learning, and the importance of keeping the two connected. She noted that teachers need knowledge, resources and practice in order to accomplish this shift to being learning-centered; that is, focused on learning. Her work discussed how the balance of power shifts and how roles for teachers and learners change in order to focus on learning. Power is shared so that the teacher and students collaborate on course policies and procedures, schedules and deadlines, and methods of learning and assesment while course content remains under the instructor's control.

Evidence on Best Practices in Teaching and Learning in Higher Education

Several prominent educators have used their research and educational experience to provide guidance for teachers in the process of learning-centered teaching. Although some of the literature is labeled for undergraduate students, much of this information is applicable to postbaccalaureate learners as well.

Chickering and Gamson (1991) used several decades of educational research to derive seven principles of good practice in undergraduate education. They indicated that good practice:

1. encourages contacts between students and faculty,

2. develops reciprocity and cooperation among students,

3. encourages active learning,

4. gives prompt feedback,

5. emphasizes time on task,

6. communicates high expectations, and

7. respects diverse talents and ways of learning.

Chickering and Ehrmann (1996) indicated that new communication and information technologies should be used in ways that are consistent with the original seven guidelines. They noted that any instructional strategy can be supported by a number of technologies and any one technology can be used to support different instructional strategies. For example, asynchronous communication via computer encourages students and faculty to engage in ongoing and multiple conversations, reflections, discourses, and responses about learning.

Evidence on Using Online Learning Environments

Virtual Learning Environments (VLEs) have assumed an important role in higher education. Also known as Learning Management Systems (LMSs) and Content Management Systems (CMSs), Virtual Learning Environments (VLEs) are learning management software systems that synthesize the functions of computer-mediated communications software and online methods of delivering course materials (Britain & Liber, 2004). Important reasons given for large-scale investment in web-based technologies are their potential to enhance teaching and learning (Jenkins, Browne, & Armitage, 2001), to encourage the development of learner-centered, independent learning (Pahl, 2003), and to foster a deep approach to learning (Collis, 1997).

Hundreds of studies were undertaken in the 1990s comparing face-to-face teaching and learning with the use of VLEs. In almost every study, no significant difference was found in student outcomes (Russell, 2001).

Deep Learning and Online Learning Environments

Several studies explored the relationship between student learning approaches or types of students and their use of VLEs. Tait, Entwistle, and McCune (1998) examined whether students' approach to learning affects their perception of the value of the VLE. They concluded that students who adopt a deep approach to learning (learning both the facts and the underlying principles) show a preference for independent study and perceive positively the use of the VLE. On the other hand, students who have a surface approach (rote learning of facts) complained about lack of time and did not complete the online tasks that were set (Jelfs & Colburn, 2002). A similar study found a negative correlation between a surface approach and the rating of the VLE (Enjelvin & Sutton, 2004).

In a study designed to determine whether VLE use demonstrates a deep approach to learning, Gibbs (1999) reported higher deep learning scores for online discussion participants versus nonparticipants as well as higher scores by strategic learners who combined elements of both deep and surface learning to complete tasks efficiently while attending to grade criteria in order to perform well. Strategic learners demonstrated their approach by their choice of online activities, which required flexibility in learning and organizational skills. Hoskins and van Hooff (2005) reported that the strategic approach is associated with more extended use of discussion boards. In the most recent study to date around deep learning, Mimirinis and Bhattacharya (2007) found that students appreciate the VLE as a learning support mechanism with a particular emphasis on flexibility and independent learning. They found a significant correlation between the strategic approach and use of the VLE to understand the meaning of concepts. This is consistent with findings from previous studies indicating that students with a strategic approach are inclined to participate more actively in a VLE (Gibbs, 1999). A deep approach to learning correlates slightly with willingness to attend to other modules on the VLE and also with a preference for face-to-face contact with a teacher rather than facilitation of learning through the VLE, suggesting that a blended approach to learning might be most effective (Mimirinis & Bhattacharya). In contrast, the scores on the surface approach scale demonstrated a slightly positive correlation with the prospect of their teacher being replaced by a VLE.

Several factors are believed to contribute to the current high levels of positive perceptions of VLEs by students. Development of a new generation of students with increased competency in instructional technology skills and provision of efficient technical support by educational institutions eliminate the previous frustration caused by lack of computer knowledge and low quality service, often reported as discouraging factors in earlier usability evaluations (Storey, Phillips, Maczewski, & Wang, 2002). Mimirinis and Bhattacharya (2007) also proposed that if the VLE is an integral part of the learning process, then a greater sense of responsibility is imposed on students, who realize that successful use of it is part of their overall success.

Design and Practice for Deep Learning Using Online Learning Environments

VLEs are shaped in many ways and most importantly by their designers. VLEs are not value-free (McNaught & Lam, 2005) in that specific values are inherent not only in their design philosophy, but also in their implementation and use. If the benefits of deep learning in a conventional teaching context apply to an online learning environment, then the design and appropriate practice may help motivate students and promote deep learning through appropriate use of VLEs. In this respect, certain parameters need to be acknowledged.

The advantages of technologies that enable collaboration, inquiry and flexibility have been discussed extensively (Hakkarainen, Lipponen, & Jaarvela, 2002; Jonassen & Kwon, 2001). The role that meaningful activities could play in engaging students needs to be emphasized. Jonassen and Kwon (2001) and Jonassen (2002) identified the following elements of a learning environment that promote meaningful learning: active, constructive, collaborative, intentional, complex, contextual, conversational, and reflective. Certain aspects of this categorization, such as the complexity of the learning environment, may be particularly useful if deep learning is to be encouraged.

Excessive workload can lead to undesired approaches to learning and poor learning outcomes (Ramsden & Entwistle, 1981). Lynch (2002) noted the danger of providing students with too many hyperlinks, resources, multimedia or other materials within the VLE. An excessive list of materials could hinder students' effort to make an understanding of the learning process and thus reproduce a surface approach. The principle of supply and demand may also be applied in this case; hyperlinks and other resources could be provided according to students' requirements and may need to correspond to their progress (Lynch, 2005; Mimirinis & Bhattacharya, 2007).

Student collaboration and communication through the use of computer-mediated communication (CMC) tools can play a crucial role in the development of a deep approach to learning. Online learning communities and networks of learners should be an aspect of all subjects using a VLE mode of delivery. Focused discussion groups and groups of people working toward common goals are practices that encourage deep learning (Berge, 1997; Lynch, 2002; Mimirinis & Bhattacharya, 2007).

Evidence on Aspects of Teaching and Learning in Nursing Education

Faculty operate within a curricular framework, which for OHSU School of Nursing is characterized by the competency and outcome statements of the various programs. The focus of this section is a brief overview of areas related to how nursing students learn or develop. We used two criteria for including the areas:

- Area is named in OHSU School of Nursing competencies and/or program outcomes, and
- A systematic integrative review of the literature or other body of evidence is available on teaching and learning in that area in nursing education

Teaching Clinical Judgment

Clinical judgment is case-based, contextually bound, interpretive reasoning (Tanner, 2006). It is one component of clinical thinking, the other component being decision-making. Clinical judgment is different from critical thinking, which has been defined as the capability to analyze assumptions, challenge the status quo, recognize limitations in health care, and take action to improve it (Ford & Profetto-McGrath, 1994). Critical thinking involves instrumental application of scientifically based knowledge to the resolution of problems, as exemplified by the nursing process. Two decades of research on critical thinking indicate the following:

- Critical thinking is a shorthand umbrella term, connoting many activities related to good thinking (Walsh & Seldomridge, 2006).
- Critical thinking and clinical thinking (i.e., decision making, clinical judgment) are different constructs, and the evidence does not support a relationship between these skills (Brunt, 2006; Hicks, 2001; Kintgen-Andrews, 1991; Staib, 2003).
- Research has not demonstrated a significant improvement in critical thinking as an outcome of nursing education. In fact, a number of studies have demonstrated substantial declines in critical thinking from beginning to end of nursing education programs (Staib, 2003).
- There is no demonstrated relationship between critical thinking and patient outcomes (Fesler-Birch, 2005).

A substantial body of research indicates that nurses in practice use the reasoning process we call clinical judgment, rather than the problem-solving approach of critical thinking (Tanner, 1998). Given that clinical judgment is case-based, contextually bound, interpretive reasoning, deep background knowledge is essential for setting up expectations of what will be seen in each clinical case, for noticing the unexpected, for considering plausible interpretations, for collecting reasonable evidence, and for choosing the best course of action. Clinical judgment always occurs in the context of the particular patient, a deep understanding of the patient's experience, preferences and values, within the ethical standards of the discipline. It takes account of the uncertainty, the unpredicted but potentially significant variables, and the process of change over time (Benner, Hooper-Kyriakidis, & Stannard, 1999; Benner, Tanner, & Chesla, 1996; Montgomery, 2006; Tanner, 2006).

An understanding of this clinical thinking has profound implications for our educational practices and demands new approaches to clinical education. For example, where nursing process and the nursing care plan decontextualize nursing judgments, emphasizing scientific rationale, teaching to clinical judgment emphasizes the narrative nature of reasoning, coaching students in the consideration of the general rule in relation to the particular case. Knowledge of clinical thinking encourages focus on educational strategies, such as case-based instructional approaches and provide guidance for simulation, group and online discussion, large-group didactic learning, and additional tools and strategies discussed later.

Teaching Reflective Practice

A review of literature by Kuiper and Pesut (2004) concluded that it is possible to help students learn reflective thinking skills, but the degree of change in reflective skills is a function of both the individual student and the amount and kind of support from teachers. Commonly used models of reflective practice include those of Mezirow (1974) and Argyris and Schön (1992). In studies applying these models, the majority of students used only lower levels of reflection, not reaching higher levels that include such outcomes as assessment of the need for further learning, or recognizing that a change in perspective is needed, or that routines they are using are not adequate. Prompts from teachers help improve student performance. As Kuiper and Pesut pointed out, "A confounding variable that influences the acquisition and development of reflective thinking is the perception of the student-teacher relationship. . . . Sharing experiences with peers and faculty in a nonjudgmental supportive milieu seems to become an essential aspect of the reflective process" (pp. 385-386).

Kuiper and Pesut also stated that "competent clinical reasoning requires a carefully constructed design, and strategies that prompt guided reflection by a mentor who makes the process meaningful, ties it to experiences, and remains available throughout learning. Clinical reasoning objectives and outcomes can be achieved with focused self-regulated learning strategies. Such strategies provide structure and are stimuli that guide reflection in the contexts of diverse experiences and individual learning styles" (p. 386) Their review of literature concludes that "Evidence suggests that investment in reflection has benefits for learning as it assists in integrating theory with practice, promotes intellectual growth, develops skills that make practitioners more confident, and fosters responsibility and accountability" (p. 386).

In a literature review on reflective practice, Mantzoukas (2008, p. 220) identified a series of steps that can guide student learning of reflective practice. These include:

1. Describing or framing of feelings, situations and context;

2. Analyzing and evaluating the situation by using various types of knowledge;

3. Verbalizing understandings, drawing conclusions and developing a hypothesis or an action plan about the specific situation;

4. Implementing the action plan; and

5. Evaluating the outcomes of the action plan and integrating the unique situation with other types of knowledge and experiences.

Teaching Evidence-Based Practice

Evidence-based practice (EBP) is a means for approaching clinical problems that represents the "conscientious use of current best evidence" (Sackett, Straus, Richardson, Rosenberg, & Haynes, 2000, as quoted in Melnyk & Fineout-Overholt, 2005, p. 6). Ingersoll (2000) furthered that definition to characterize evidence-based nursing as the conscientious, explicit and judicious use of theory-derived, research-based information in making decisions about care delivery systems and in consideration of internal and external consumer needs and preferences. Melnyk and Fineout-Overholt added the following components to the definition:

- a systematic search for and critical appraisal of the most relevant evidence to answer a burning clinical question,
- one's own clinical expertise, and
- patient preferences and values.

Fineout-Overholt, Cox, Robbins, and Gray (2005) noted that at least two models presenting comprehensive plans for teaching and developing evidence users are available. However, these authors indicated that current evidence supporting the effectiveness of teaching EBP lacks quality. Two outcomes from research on teaching EBP in health professions do seem to have importance. First, several studies strongly suggested that seminars focusing on specific EBP skills can measurably improve those skills (Bennett et al., 1987; Green & Ellis, 1997; Linzer, Brown, Frazier, DeLong, & Siegal, 1988; Norman & Shannon, 1998; Seelig, 1991). Some examples of targeted EBP skills include learning to ask searchable questions, search the health care databases and literature, and read health care research critically. A second outcome from research supports the notion that curricula are most successful in helping students to become users of research when EBP principles are utilized in different settings and formats (e.g., classroom, clinical setting) and presented in a variety of ways (e.g., journal club, morning report) (Norman & Shannon, 1998; Sackett & Parks, 1998). In other words, a pervasive culture appears to provide the most successful preparation in EBP for health care students. Part of this culture should include mentoring (Morrison-Beedy, Aronowitz, Dyne, & Mkandawire, 2001). The evidence about curriculum supports an early introduction to research and its integration throughout the curriculum rather than placing all EBP principles into a single research course.

Many systematic reviews are available that focus on a particular clinical problem, but none were found that address the effective teaching of evidence-based practice to students. Much more research needs to be done to discover and evaluate the most effective ways of teaching students to become effective EBP users.

Teaching Ethical Practice

Articles on ethics instruction in professional education consistently cited the need to supplement classroom instruction on ethical concepts and principles with faculty role modeling and, finally, practical application. Suggested application of content uses case scenarios and real-life learning situations.

Aiken and Cataleno (1994) stated that students acquire values in nursing both directly and indirectly. Direct acquisition first takes place in lecture or small group discussions and through readings that introduce models for analysis and decision-making, relevant codes of ethics, basic principles, and essential values of the discipline. Secondly, case-based scenarios in small group seminars apply ethical and professional values to practice situations. Methods of high-level questioning promote Bloom's levels of analysis and evaluation (Boswell, 2005; Weaver & Morse, 2006). Preparing key questions based on classroom learning and required readings allows faculty to focus on encouraging reflective thinking in students. Socratic questioning was recommended to help the student acquire ethical sensitivity and promote critical decision-making. Questions having no right or wrong answer enhance self-reflection and sensitivity (Candela, Dalley, & Benzel-Lindley, 2006). Peers introduce diversity to challenge student reflection further. Students then are ready to apply these concepts to clinical situations with the direct help of faculty on their clinical units or in post conference. Students also learn ethical practice indirectly from faculty role modeling. Thus, it is suggested that faculty periodically reflect on their own values and ethical stance to prevent bias (Baxter & Boblin, 2007; Beckett, Gilbertson, & Greenwood, 2007).

Most of the articles on ethics instruction were descriptive, citing methods to teach ethics based on solid teaching-learning principles and conceptual models of ethical decision-making. No integrative reviews were found. A few studies provided evidence to support the methods described. Corey, Corey, and Callanan (2005) discussed the use of computer scenarios demonstrating ethical decision-making in the clinical setting. These scenarios were used for discussion and subsequent teaching in small group seminars. These authors also promoted the use of reaction papers, role play, and guest speakers. Their methods were evaluated positively through students' written comments. Leners, Roehrs, and Piccone (2006) studied student learning of professional values through the methods of lecture, case-based practice examples, and clinical application. Using a scale to measure student professional values at semester one and again after semester five, Leners et al. found that most student nurses' values scores significantly increased over the five-semester BSN program.

Teaching Cultural Competence

The American Association of Colleges of Nursing (2008) articulates five cultural competencies for baccalaureate nursing education, which are the abilities to:
- apply knowledge of social and cultural factors that affect nursing and health care across multiple contexts;
- use relevant data sources and best evidence in providing culturally competent care;

- promote achievement of safe and quality outcomes of care for diverse populations;
- advocate for social justice, including commitment to the health of vulnerable populations and the elimination of health disparities; and
- participate in continuous cultural competence development.

An integrative review of teaching cultural competence in nursing was not found to date, however, a systematic review of the literature from the Joanna Briggs Institute on development of cultural competence in the health care workforce provided clear recommendations for embedding this learning into nursing education (Pearson et al., 2007). These recommendations focused on developing knowledge and understanding of minority groups as well as skill in communication, flexibility and openness. In addition, the literature suggested that the following elements should be included when teaching cultural competence (Byrne, Weddle, Davis, & McGinnis, 2003; Campinha-Bacote, 1999; Greene, 1993; Schim, Doorenbos, & Borse, 2005):

- various definitions of cultural competence and philosophical inquiries into its nature;
- definitions and discussions of related terms (such as being inclusionary, multicultural, race, color, diversity, white privilege);
- assessments to determine cultural competence;
- strategies to remove cultural bias from instructional materials;
- facts about numbers of diverse patients and models to increase cultural competence in health care; and
- consideration of diversity as a socio-eco-political feature of higher education.

The Institute of Medicine (2004) asserted that greater racial and ethnic diversity among health professionals would improve the access to and quality of health care for all Americans. However, recent reports indicated that we have made few gains in recruiting and retaining a more ethnically diverse workforce (Sullivan Commission, 2005). While minority group representation is rapidly approaching 33 percent of the US population, today's nursing students certainly do not mirror this. Only 5.4 percent of all RNs are men and only 12.3 percent of RNs represent racial or ethnic minority groups, according to the 2000 National Sample Survey of Registered Nurses, prepared by the federal Division of Nursing within the Bureau of Health Professions (AACN, 2001). The systematic review by Pearson et al. (2007) mentioned previously notes the importance of recruiting and retaining a diverse workforce as a key component of delivering culturally competent care.

Schim and colleagues (2005) used the term culturally congruent care, which they described as follows: "Culturally congruent care occurs when providers and recipients of health services come together with an attitude of cultural humility and respect. They can then negotiate mutually satisfactory strategies to address health promotion, disease prevention, restoration of health, or a 'good death', as defined by the person needing care. For culturally congruent care to occur, providers need a knowledge base, attitudinal framework, and skill set to appreciate, accommodate, and negotiate cultural and individual variations in beliefs, values, lifestyles, education and the myriad elements that comprise cultural context" (p. 354). This description embodies the components of cultural competence that the teacher of nursing must consider when planning learning experience for students to develop this component of professional nursing practice. The desired outcome is that students learn how to incorporate their personal knowledge of cultural diversity, their awareness of other peoples and their cultures, and their sensitivity to that knowledge into their practice behaviors.

Teaching Interprofessional Collaboration

Interprofessional collaboration was noted as an essential outcome by both the American Association of Colleges of Nursing (1996, 1998) and the Accreditation Council for Graduate Medical Education (ACGME, 1999). In 2003, the Institute of Medicine recommended interprofessional education (IPE) as one of five recommendations to improve collaboration and hence, patient safety. There were a few early adopters (Mitchell, Stegbauer, & Watson, 2005), but the momentum is just beginning to build.

A recent review focused entirely on the pedagogy of IPE (Payler, Meyer, & Humphris, 2008). The authors used the literature when there was mention of interprofessional teaching strategies and learning as well as evaluation. The approaches fell into several categories: IPE with specific client groups, problem-based IPE, practice-based IPE, and collaborative learning approaches. Because of the complexity involved in IPE, the literature is missing detailed descriptions or evidence to support these approaches. Little consensus of approach was noted, except that IPE is complex and requires excellent facilitation to promote equity and respect. The conclusion of the review was that IPE pedagogy is very new, which compounds the difficulty of evaluation, and there is little evidence for various pedagogies or evaluation tools used. The primary evaluation focus has been self-evaluated attitudinal changes. More descriptive pedagogical approaches and evidence-based evaluation strategies are needed.

The Carnegie Foundation for the Advancement of Teaching sponsored the Preparation for the Professions Program, a comparative study of professional education. The purposes of the study were to identify the best practices for preparing professionals in nursing (Benner, Sutphen, Leonard, & Day, 2010), medicine (Cooke, Irby, O'Brien, & Shulman, 2010), law (Sullivan, Colby, Wegner, 2007), engineering (Sheppard, Macatangay, Colby, & Sullivan, 2008), and clergy (Foster, Dahill, Golemon, Tolentino, 2005) and to help each to understand the perspectives of the other, particularly where there are similarities. This research may provide implications for interprofessional health education in the future.

Teaching Self-Directed Learning

The literature on self-directed learning supports the idea that it is important for nurses to have the skills to seek, analyze, and use information effectively, and that nursing education can play an important role in aiding students to acquire these skills (Lunyk-Child et al., 2001; Majumdar, 1996). Rampogus (1988) suggested that learning how to learn is an essential and critical component in the education of student nurses. Kell and Van Deursen (2002) contended that teachers should ensure that students acquire self-directed learning skills that can be transferred from their education to the work situation.

Studies in other fields suggested that specialist teachers can influence students' self-direction. A quantitative study involving medical students found that groups taught by "content-expert" teachers produced twice as many learning issues for self-directed learning as students taught by "non-content-expert" teachers (Eagle, Harasym, & Mandlin, 1992). Similarly, another study found that medical students taught by experts spent significantly more time on self-directed learning than those taught by non-experts (Schmidt, Van Der Arend, Moust, Kokx, & Boon, 1993). Dolmans and colleagues (2002) contended that ideally a teacher should be both an expert in the subject being taught and an expert in facilitating learning. This has implications for nursing education, in that it suggests the need for ongoing faculty and clinical preceptor development within nursing specialties and also for ensuring that nurses engaged in teaching understand how people learn.

Numerous articles described the implementation of self-directed learning within nursing programs (Armstrong, 1986; DeSilets, 1986; Dyck, 1986; Hamilton

& Gregor, 1986; Jenkins, Carlson, & Herrick, 1998; Majumdar, 1996; Weinberg & Stone-Griffith, 1992). It is beyond the scope of this review to explore each of these individually. These articles were all descriptive in nature, either suggesting ways of developing self-directed learning modules or describing their actual use. All of the documented approaches to self-directed learning appear to involve several stages: assessment (of the environment, readiness for self-direction, learning needs, resources); planning; implementing; and evaluating. These reflected the stages put forward by Knowles (1975) in setting up a student-centered learning environment: creating a climate for learning, identifying learning needs and learning resources, carrying out the learning activity, evaluating learning, and identifying future needs.

The application of self-directed learning is not without its problems. In self-directed learning, the responsibility for decisions rests with the individual student and the impact of this change in responsibility cannot be underestimated (Iwasiw, 1987). Indeed, many authors identified that students initially experience anxiety and fear about self-directed learning and report the need for an introduction to the concept (Lunyk-Child et al., 2001; Miflin, Campbell, & Price, 2000; Nolan, & Nolan, 1997; Prociuk, 1990). Kocaman, Dicle, and Ugur (2009) found that becoming a self-directed learner is a maturational process, with student perceptions of their own readiness increasing over time.

Nolan and Nolan (1997) advanced a cooperative model for implementation of self-directed learning. They suggested that students may find self-directed learning stressful and require support and direction, particularly during the early stages of their course. In a study of teachers' and students' perceptions of self-directed learning, Lunyk-Child et al. (2001) found that students undergo a transformation that begins with negative feelings (e.g., confusion, frustration, dissatisfaction) and ends with confidence and skill for self-direction. During this transformation, teachers need to provide learner support.

Learner support can take the form of instruction in the self-directed learning process. In discussing the role of nurse teachers in self-directed learning, Iwasiw (1987) argued that students should receive a cognitive understanding of the self-directed learning process before they can be expected to engage in it. Knowles (1980) acknowledged that adults may be unused to self-directed learning and may initially find it problematic. Indeed, in Prociuk's (1990) study, 61 percent of respondents agreed with the statement "In retrospect, I needed an introduction to the self-directed learning process at the beginning of my orientation programme." This need for instruction was confirmed by Hewitt-Taylor (2001) in a study of self-directed learning in pediatric intensive care nursing, where both students and teachers considered that self-directed learning required some guidelines in order to be successful.

Teaching Therapeutic Communication and Relationship Skills

A multitude of books and articles on communication skills and the therapeutic relationship in nursing all assert the importance of good communication skills to nursing practice. The teaching methods that are described are based on communication theory and models using principles of teaching-learning; however, there were very few research studies on the best method to teach communication and relationship skills. The consensus is that such skills are learned through didactic learning of communication models, communication skills, core relationship dimensions and then by planning, rehearsing and practicing. Modeling by faculty, clinical agency preceptors, and other role models influences the nursing student indirectly.

In a pilot study, Kluge and Glick (2006) found that using a video-interactive, computer-based, challenge-response-record-evaluate method was an effective way to develop communication skills. In a study designed to test the Simulated Client Interview Rating Scale (SCIRS), Arthur (1999) used the scale after an intensive training in Rollnick and Miller's Motivational Interviewing and found improvement in the students' performance.

Ferrari (2006) found consensus about the importance of experiential learning, and that confidence in communication skills could be improved with training using discussions, role play and videos. His qualitative study supported academic education, practice, and reflection as important to bridge the gap between theory and practice. The students he studied also valued experiential methods used in seminars such as case studies, role play, and group discussion.

No integrative reviews were found. One systematic review of the literature (Chant, Jenkinson, Randle, & Russell, 2002) examined 200 relevant articles but found difficulties in comparing studies due to overlap in the definition of the terms communication skills and interpersonal skills. Based on their literature review, the authors identified variability in skills taught, including deficient training in telephone, computer, and media communication and to special populations (e.g., elderly, disabled, hearing impaired, mentally ill). Based on the idea that exposure to role modeling increases competence, the authors suggested that changes are needed in education and practice to value communication equally with physical care and task completion so that learning by role modeling can take place. Most importantly, they decried the lack of evaluative studies of the effectiveness of the various models for teaching therapeutic communication.

Evidence Regarding Pedagogical Strategies

The tools and strategies discussed in this section were selected because integrative reviews of evidence for their effectiveness have been published. This section is not intended to be comprehensive. The discussion focuses on clinical education, simulation, case-based learning, concept maps, group and online discussion, collaborative learning, large-group didactic learning, ways to engage students, and assessment/feedback.

Clinical Education

A position paper to provide guidance to boards of nursing for evaluating the clinical experience component of prelicensure programs was prepared by the National Council of State Boards of Nursing (NCSBN) Practice, Regulation and Education (PR&E) Committee (NCSBN, 2005). The detailed literature review and analysis in the position paper generated the following recommendations:

- Prelicensure nursing educational experiences should be across the lifespan.
- Prelicensure nursing education programs should include clinical experiences with actual patients; they might also include innovative teaching strategies that complement clinical experiences for entry into practice competency.
- Prelicensure clinical education should be supervised by qualified faculty who provide feedback and facilitate reflection.
- Faculty members should retain the responsibility of ensuring that programs have sufficient clinical experiences with actual patients to meet program outcomes.
- Additional research needs to be conducted on prelicensure nursing education programs and the development of clinical competency. (NCSBN, 2005, p. 1)

An integrative review of literature by Udlis (2008) concerning preceptorship versus traditional clinical educational experiences concluded the following:

- Preceptorship supports and nurtures the development of adaptive learning competencies.
- The preceptored environment is congruent with the learning styles of nursing students and promotes effective learning and transfer of knowledge.
- Preceptorship programs appear to support and augment professional nursing role development.
- The empirical literature does not support that preceptorship improves critical care skills or promotes critical thinking, clinical competence, or improvement in NCLEX-RN® pass rates over traditional clinical experiences. (Udlis, 2008, p.28)

Benner's (2004) model of skill acquisition and clinical judgment and Ericcson's (2004) review of deliberate practice provided significant contributions to the NCSBN's review of the theoretical background related to clinical education.

Simulation

An early systematic review of best evidence in medical education (BEME), covering three decades of literature, addressed the question, "What are the features and uses of high-fidelity medical simulations that lead to most effective learning?" (Issenberg, McGaghie, Petrusa, Gordon, & Scalese, 2005, p. 10). Although the focus was on medical education, many applications to nursing education are apparent. The strength of evidence was highest for 10 features of high-fidelity simulation, the top three of which included: (a) providing feedback (47 percent), (b) repetitive practice (39 percent), and (c) curriculum integration (25 percent). The review observed that while simulation as a training tool does not duplicate patients in real clinical settings, it certainly complements it. Noting that the current health care environment does not always provide adequate learning opportunities for students, simulation does "boost learner self-confidence and perseverance, [as well as] affective education outcomes that accompany clinical competence" (p. 24).

Since 2005, nursing research in simulation has gained momentum. A longitudinal, multisite study, cosponsored by the National League for Nursing and Laerdal (manufacturer of SimMan®), resulted in a discourse of best practices (Jeffries, 2007). A subsequent systematic review addresses teaching and learning effectiveness in nursing education through the use of high-fidelity patient simulation. Kaakinen and Arwood (2009) concluded that the paradigm shift from teaching to learning, similar to that characterized by Barr and Tagg (1995), must form the basis for simulation design in order to measure simulation's effectiveness as a learning tool.

Many recent reports of studies and best practices described effective learning through the process of debriefing the simulation (Dreifuerst, 2009; Fanning, & Gaba, 2007; Lasater, 2007a; Rudolph, Simon, Dufresne, & Raemer, 2006; Rudolph, Simon, Raemer, & Eppich, 2008). Others focused on evaluation of student learning following simulation and transfer of learning to the clinical practice setting (Cato, Lasater, & Peeples, 2009; Dillard et al., 2009; Lasater, 2007b).

In followup to Issenberg et al. (2005), Leigh (2008) reviewed studies that see high-fidelity patient simulation through the lens of students' acquisition of confidence and self-efficacy. Although Leigh concluded that human patient simulation is an effective teaching method and that students and faculty believe that simulation improves clinical performance, the literature did not conclusively support that simulation raises self-efficacy above other teaching modalities nor did it support that new grads' confidence or self-efficacy is enhanced by simulation at this time.

In addition to the features of simulation already discussed, future research should investigate the optimal ratio of simulation to clinical practice and continue to study how learning in the simulation laboratory transfers into the clinical setting. Additional research attention is needed regarding building confidence and self-efficacy in practice, whether simulation reinforces learning about enhancing quality and safe patient outcomes, and if simulation holds potential for summative evaluation.

The NCBSN (2005) position paper discussed above noted several aspects of simulation as a learning strategy. With the first point updated, it provided a summary that may guide future research:

- Simulation began as a complement, not a substitute, to clinical experiences. However, as faculty have become more confident in simulation's learning effectiveness, simulation has replaced a portion of clinical hours in many programs (Nehring, 2008).
- Simulation incorporates deliberate practice.
- Simulation provides self-paced education with safe outcomes.
- Simulation does not necessarily involve expensive equipment.
- Simulation gives students self-confidence.
- Simulation enhances team performances.
- Feedback is a key component of both simulation and clinical experiences (adapted from NCSBN, 2005, p. 8).

Case-Based Learning

Case-based instructional approaches were supported by the research literature. A literature review by Tomey (2003) indicated that "case studies apply theories and didactic content to simulations of real-life situations. With case studies, an in-depth analysis of a situation is used to illustrate class content. Learners not only apply their background knowledge, but gain new learning to solve the problem" (p. 34). Tomey concluded that "case methods or studies provide a process of participatory learning that facilitates active and reflective learning and results in the development of critical thinking and effective problem-solving skills. This develops self-directed, lifelong learners. Learners are exposed to complex situations, can discuss and debate courses of action and have the opportunity to perform. Cases help build on prior knowledge, integrate knowledge, and consider application to future situations. Cases encourage teamwork and accountability and are realistic and motivating to adult learners" (p. 37).

Concept Maps

Concept maps diagram key concepts into a framework of related propositions (Novak & Gowin, 1984). The goal of concept mapping is to assist learners in developing links from old concepts they already know to new concepts they are trying to master. Students become engaged learners by drawing connections between concepts. This process results in meaningful learning that helps students assimilate new knowledge and develop deep understanding of complex ideas (Ausbel, Novak, & Hanesian, 1978; Schuster, 2002).

Clayton (2006) presented a comprehensive review of the research literature on concept mapping in nursing education for the period up to 2004 (seven studies). Five additional studies conducted since 2004 were located through the CINAHL database, using the search term *concept mapping*. All twelve studies reported that student perceptions of the use of concept maps as a learning strategy were positive. Ten of the twelve studies used increases in student knowledge and critical thinking ability as outcome variables. Students using concept maps attained higher exam scores (Gaines, 1996; Rooda, 1994; Wheeler & Collins, 2003) and show improvements in critical thinking skills (August-Brady, 2005; Daley, Shaw, Balistrieri, Glasenapp, & Piacentine, 1999; Hicks-Moore & Pastirik, 2006; Hinck et al., 2006; Wheeler & Collins). In most of the studies, the differences were statistically significant.

August-Brady reported that students using concept maps demonstrated a significant increase in deep approach to learning and self-regulation of that learning. Hinck and colleagues demonstrated that concept mapping significantly increases student ability to see patterns and relationships for planning and evaluating nursing care. Four studies examined growth in student ability to construct concept maps and demonstrated that much practice, feedback from faculty, and participation in collaborative groups in constructing maps all increased student ability to use this learning tool and enhanced satisfaction with concept mapping as a learning strategy (Caelli, 1998; Daley et al.,1999; Hsu & Hsieh, 2005; Kinchin & Hay, 2005).

Discussion and Questioning Strategies

Appropriate use of questioning strategies by teachers can facilitate the development of critical thinking skills and decision-making ability (Boswell, 2005; Gerrish, 1992; Meleca, Schimfhauser, Witteman, & Sachs, 1981; Pond, Bradshaw, & Turner 1991). Bloom's taxonomy of the six levels of cognitive learning is a useful framework for constructing questions (Bloom, 1956; Phillips & Duke, 2001). Bloom's taxonomy progresses from knowledge (the simplest level of learning) to evaluation (the most complex level). The words used to construct a question determine the level of the answer (Russell, Comello, & Wright, 2007).

A study by Scholdra and Quiring (1973) determined what proportion of terminal objectives for clinical nursing courses in a baccalaureate nursing program were high-level objectives (analysis, synthesis, evaluation) and what level of questions were asked by teachers and students during clinical conferences. Despite the fact that stated objectives specified higher cognitive-level thinking, lower-level questions comprised 98.94 percent of the total number of questions asked by teachers and students in the clinical conferences surveyed. Similarly, several other studies found that clinical teachers tend to ask low-level questions rather than high-level questions, even though the higher level is required for deep learning (Phillips & Duke, 2001; Profetto-McGrath, Smith, Day, & Yonge, 2004; Sellappah, Hussey, Blackmore, & McMurray, 1998).

Since questioning is an integral part of teaching that can assist students in applying their knowledge (Phillips & Duke, 2001), teachers need to know how to use questioning strategies effectively. To facilitate a chain of reasoning, questions need to be asked in a logical format, either deductively or inductively (Sellappah et al., 1998). Asking questions that have more than one possible answer allows for different viewpoints and encourages students to compare problems and approaches (Oermann, 1997). Another form of questioning is focused reflection and articulation to promote clinical reasoning. Murphy (2004) described research demonstrating that students with high clinical reasoning report a high frequency of use of focused reflection and articulation. Cranton (2006) identified three types of questions as effective for increasing self-reflection and understanding of one's own and others' viewpoints:

- Content reflection questions "raise learner awareness of assumptions and beliefs" (p. 139).
- Process reflection questions "address how a person has come to hold a certain perspective" (p. 140).
- Premise reflection questions address why a person holds certain beliefs or why these beliefs are so important to the person.

Another type of questioning technique is Socratic questioning, which deeply probes or explores the meaning, justification, or logical strength of a claim, position, or line of reasoning (Paul & Heaslip, 1995). The questions investigate assumptions, viewpoints, consequences, and evidence. Asking one student to summarize the answer of another student allows the student to demonstrate that he or she was listening, had digested the information, and understood it enough to put it into his or her own words.

In addition to using these questioning techniques, it is equally important to orient the students to this type of classroom interaction. Mills (1995) suggested that provocative questions should be brief and contain only one or two issues at a time for class reflection. If a thought question is asked, time must be given for the students to think about the answer (Dillon, 1990; Mills). Providing at least 5 seconds of deliberate silence allows the students to think and encourages thought. Elliot (1996) argued that waiting even as long as 10 seconds allows the students time to think about possibilities.

Students' answers to questions posed by their teachers provide potentially useful feedback and the questions that students ask reflect their progress in the course. According to Lozano (2001), "Answering questions may show the instructor that the student remembers the answer to a question or problem, but asking questions shows that students are actively thinking" (p. 25).

Weimer (2002) and Brookfield and Preskill (1999) wrote about the role of discussion in engaging the students, an effective and necessary practice in the focus on the learner. Both of these processes of student-teacher engagement, discussion and questioning strategies, are relevant to the development of critical thinking and clinical judgment.

Collaborative Learning

In collaborative learning, the faculty member becomes a facilitator rather than a transmitter of learning (Barkley, Cross, & Major, 2004; Matthews, Cooper, Davidson, & Hawkes, 1995). While varied in form, collaborative learning experiences emphasize interdependence in achieving learning outcomes (Davidson, 1994; Freeth & Reeves, 2004; Panitz, 2004).

According to Vygotsky (1978), students are capable of performing at higher intellectual levels when asked to work in collaborative situations than when asked to work individually. Group diversity in terms of knowledge and experience contributes positively to the learning process. Bruner (1985) contended that cooperative learning methods improve problem-solving strategies because the students are confronted with different interpretations of the given situation. The peer support system makes it possible for the learner to internalize both external knowledge and critical thinking skills and to convert them into tools for intellectual functioning.

No integrative review of research on effectiveness of collaborative learning was found. Gokhale (1995) studied the impact of collaborative learning on critical thinking in higher education students. She found collaborative learning fosters the development of critical thinking through discussion, clarification of ideas, and evaluation of others' ideas.

Schön (1987) described collaborative learning as an integral part of the reflective process. He stated that the role and behavior of the teacher as coach is of prime importance in the success of reflective practice and collaboration of the learners. Bruffee (1993) used computer-mediated communications (CMC) in a supportive environment that allowed students to engage in reflective peer discussions on clinical practice and professional issues. Oliver and Naidu (1997) also used CMC to assist students to apply their content knowledge to medical-surgical nursing practice. Through collaborative reflection in discussion forums and shared learning logs, students became more adept at making the links between professional practice and their formal education.

Large-Group Didactic Learning

No integrative review of large-group didactic learning has been located. Both Bain (2004) and Weimer (2002) emphasized the importance of teacher attitude and approach rather than use of specific techniques in effective large-group didactic learning. Through extensive research on outstanding college teachers, Bain found that outstanding teachers in various disciplines possess similar qualities and attitudes that are evident in effective large-group didactic learning and in other teaching environments. These teachers:

- Are experts in their fields, know how to explain complex subjects clearly, and can think metacognitively;
- Conceptualize learning as a process wherein students construct an understanding rather than receive knowledge; foster intrinsic motivators; and engage students' reasoning abilities;
- Focus first on student learning outcomes, designing learning experiences to foster those outcomes;
- Stimulate high achievement by treating each student as unique, believing in students' ability to achieve, setting high standards, promoting intellectual excitement and curiosity, providing opportunity to apply learning to meaningful problems, allowing students to set authentic goals, and assisting them to achieve them;
- Create a critical learning environment in which students confront engaging problems, feel a sense of control, work collaboratively with others, and receive feedback separately from summative evaluation of their efforts;
- Capture students' attention and keep it for the duration of the class session by moving from familiar topics to new and challenging ones;
- Encourage learning outside the classroom; create diverse learning experiences; create a conversation in the classroom; use warm, inviting language; give clear explanations; and promote participation in discussions;
- Seek commitment from students, believe that students want to learn, invest in them to help them learn, and treat them with fairness and compassion;
- Use assessment to help students learn rather than simply to evaluate their work;
- Have a systematic program to evaluate their own teaching, do not blame students for their own difficulties, and have a strong commitment to the academic community.

These characteristics of outstanding teachers enable them to spark learning in large-group didactic settings that makes a long-term difference in their students' ability to reason with the concepts and information they encountered in class (Bain, 2004; Weimer, 2002), echoing the work of Bransford, Brown, and Cocking (2004) on how people learn, as well as illustrating the best practices in teaching and learning enumerated by Chickering and Gamson (1991).

Faculty Development and Evaluation

Background

Within the context of a program of nursing education, the strategic plan and faculty governance structure should support both faculty development and evaluation of teaching effectiveness. The missions of teaching, research, and practice should be equally valued. Accepting the significance of multiple, complex missions is consonant with the tenets of professional accountability as well as a full acknowledgment of the scholarship with which teaching must be approached in a research university. Boyer (1990) expressed this principle clearly when he said that the work of the scholar "becomes consequential only as it is understood by others" (p. 23). Scholarship understood by others does not exist in traditional faculty mission categories, because it is an act of knowledge transformation. Some examples of scholarship translated to increase understanding in students are beginning to appear in the literature (Bekemeier & Butterfield, 2005; Boutain, 2005). The following sections consider faculty development and faculty evaluation of teaching separately, although they should be integrated in their implementation.

Faculty Development

Faculty development in the education mission is a long-term process of assisting faculty as they transform their teaching. In so doing, the process should foster faculty retention, continued professional growth, and promotion. Faculty development should encompass professional growth in all the missions at all levels. The goals for faculty development in teaching scholarship should:

- promote active engagement with the substance of nursing for both students and faculty;
- foster reflection on that engagement and its outcomes while increasing student understanding of the content and processes, ethical reasoning and

clinical judgment that underlie the practice of nursing.

Faculty development includes components that focus on strategies to promote (a) successful integration into the faculty role in the institution, including a well-defined orientation with information about professional growth and guidelines for promotion (Morin & Ashton, 2004); (b) ongoing opportunities to improve teaching; (c) a culture that supports and recognizes scholarship in teaching; and (d) structures that provide for formal career development (Boyer, 1990; Peters & Boylston, 2006; Weimer, 2002). In addition, faculty development should be considered within the range of lifelong learning and be intentional, planned, and proactive. Reflective practice (Schön, 1987; Tanner, 2006) is an integral component of faculty development, both for continued personal growth and improvement as well as practicing and modeling what faculty expect of students.

In the context of lifelong learning, teaching excellence is a natural outgrowth of faculty development (Hesketh et al., 2001; Noone & Swenson, 2001), fostering reflection and curiosity, and providing opportunities to satisfy inquisitiveness. These qualities should promote increasing excellence. As described earlier, teaching excellence is learner-centered (Weimer, 2002).

Formation and sustenance of community among colleagues is a critical element of faculty development (Palmer, 1998), particularly for faculty who are new to academia and all faculty who are interested in the scholarship of teaching (Shulman, 2004). Nurture in the form of mentoring at all levels (National League for Nursing [NLN], 2006a; Sigma Theta Tau, 2006), but especially among the least experienced, should be paramount in faculty development planning. Mentorship is a reciprocal process in which both the mentor and the mentee learn. Mentoring faculty and building community may be especially important retention strategies, in view of the nursing faculty shortage (Tanner, 2001), both nationally and statewide. Retaining and developing a consistent, long-term community of faculty should take precedence over short-term hiring to fill an acute need.

Faculty Evaluation

Faculty evaluation is intended to be a formative process (Bransford, Brown, & Cocking, 2004), allowing faculty to learn and grow from the process and to determine what changes are best instituted to enhance learning for themselves and their students. Evaluation should demonstrate continued growth or development over time, an important correlation of evaluation with faculty development. In addition, faculty evaluation should be an efficient process, with multiple points of evidence predetermined by the community of faculty, a clear, collegial, and cumulative process without being onerous (Buckingham & Coffman, 2004), and one that supports faculty's long-term goals as well as the university and program's vision and mission.

Faculty evaluation most often is based on identified criteria; nearly all academic institutions currently use those proffered by Boyer (1990), requiring faculty to provide evidence of the specified criteria. Some may argue that evaluation should root itself only in evidence (Johnson & Ryan, 2000) that is traditionally measurable or observable, but newer literature suggests expansion of the typical sources of evidence (Knapper, 2001). For example, a menu of evaluation options for the annual review could provide triangulation of the evidence (e.g., student, self, peer) for teaching effectiveness. Questions for consideration regarding faculty evaluation include: (a) should external review be an option? (b) what are the criteria for evaluators? and (c) are expectations clearly defined and/or individualized?

Faculty evaluation includes the annual review as well as review for promotion and/or tenure. Traditionally, the evidence of teaching excellence for the annual review has been based on student evaluations, amplified by feedback from the program director (Hewson & Little, 1998). Anecdotal reports from numerous programs note that when programs change to online student evaluations, the number of completed evaluations diminishes dramatically. Efforts should focus on improvement of the completion rate through incentives, and upgrading the quality of the information gleaned from student evaluations.

The process for promotion and tenure is another form of evaluation. The annual evaluation review should be a valid and important step to assist faculty toward their long-term goals, such as supporting their efforts in the promotion and tenure process (Furney et al., 2001; Newman & Peile, 2002). Faculty should be oriented to the promotion and tenure process early in their academic careers and have opportunities for career planning and mentorship in order to work toward promotion and/or tenure. The process needs to be transparent so that faculty can effectively plan their career trajectories.

In order to retain faculty and foster growth, there should be a process of recognition for achievement of faculty at all levels, regardless of eligibility for promotion. As faculty progress in their teaching excellence and take on additional scholarly activity, such as writing for peer-reviewed journals, leadership within the curriculum, or speaking at conferences, they should be recognized for their continued growth and contributions. Successful completion of the National League for Nursing Certification Exam (NLN, 2005) or matriculation through post-master's education should be recognized.

Summary

Research on learning indicates that students construct their learning based on what they know. In order to develop competence in an area of inquiry, they need a deep knowledge base and conceptual frameworks to organize their knowledge. Students take control of their own learning when they reflect on and monitor their own progress. Best practices in teaching and learning in higher education are presented in the seven principles delineated by Chickering and Gamson (1991), which are to: encourage contacts between students and faculty, develop reciprocity and cooperation among students, encourage active learning, give prompt feedback, emphasize time on task, communicate high expectations, and respect diverse talents and ways of learning. These best practices can be employed in face-to-face and online learning environments.

Nursing faculty must utilize effective methods when teaching important aspects of nursing practice such as clinical judgment, reflective thinking skills, evidence-based practice, and self-directed learning. Clinical judgment (case-based, contextually bound, interpretive reasoning) and decision-making are the two components of clinical thinking. Knowledge of the nature of clinical thinking can guide the use of pedagogical strategies. Students learn reflective thinking skills most effectively when faculty provide prompts that stimulate reflection at a high level and provide ongoing mentorship. Teaching evidence-based practice appears to be most effective when evidence-based practice principles are used in different settings and formats rather than confined to one setting or course. Research on teaching ethical practice supports the use of case-based scenarios and questions that have no right or wrong answers in order to enhance self-reflection. The research on teaching self-directed learning indicates that students may find self-directed learning stressful and may require support and direction in the early stages.

Research literature does not provide evidence regarding the most effective ways to teach some important aspects of nursing practice, including cultural competence, interdisciplinary collaboration, and therapeutic communication and relationship skills. Literature on cultural competence provides definitions and identifies components that need to be taught, but does not provide much evidence regarding effective ways to teach this important aspect of professional nursing practice. Interdisciplinary collaboration is noted as an essential outcome of education, but research evidence to support effective ways of teaching it is lacking. Finally, despite the widely held belief that therapeutic communication and relationship skills are learned through experiential learning, evaluation studies are needed.

The pedagogical strategies that were discussed in this monograph are supported by integrative reviews or extensive research providing evidence for their effectiveness. These strategies include clinical education, high-fidelity simulation as a complement to clinical experiences, case-based participatory learning, concept-mapping to develop links between familiar and unfamiliar concepts, discussion and questioning strategies that promote deep learning, collaborative learning in which faculty serve as coaches, and large-group didactic learning. Among other characteristics, faculty who are effective in large-group didactic learning are experts in their fields, believe that students must learn to use facts simultaneously with learning the facts themselves, focus on student learning outcomes and design learning experiences to foster those outcomes, stimulate high achievement, and have a systematic program to evaluate their own teaching.

Faculty development and evaluation of teaching effectiveness support best practices in teaching and learning and should be integrated in their application. Viewed in the context of lifelong learning, faculty development promotes learner-based teaching excellence and is nurtured by formation and sustenance of community among colleagues. Faculty evaluation is best viewed as a formative process that allows faculty to learn and grow from the process and optimally provides multiple points of evidence based on identified criteria that encompass best practices in teaching and learning.

References

Accreditation Council for Graduate Medical Education (ACGME). (1999). ACGME general competencies, version 1.3. Retrieved from http://www.acgme.org/outcome/comp/compMin.asp

Aiken, T. D., & Cataleno, J. T. (1994). *Legal, ethical and political issues in nursing.* Philadelphia: F. A. Davis.

American Association of Colleges of Nursing. (1996). *The essentials of master's education for advanced practice nursing.* Washington, DC: Author.

American Association of Colleges of Nursing. (1998). *The essentials of baccalaureate education for nursing.* Washington, DC: Author.

American Association of Colleges of Nursing. (2001). Issue bulletin: *Effective strategies for increasing diversity in nursing programs.* Retrieved from http://www.aacn.nche.edu/Publications/issues/dec01.htm

American Association of Colleges of Nursing. (2008). *Cultural competency in baccalaureate nursing education.* Retrieved from http://www.aacn.nche.edu/Education/pdf/competency.pdf

Argyris, C., & Schön, D. A. (1992). *Theory in practice: Increasing professional effectiveness.* San Francisco: Jossey-Bass.

Armstrong, M. (1986). Self-directed learning about computers and computers for self-directed learning. *Journal of Continuing Education in Nursing, 17*(3), 84-86.

Arthur, D. (1999). Assessing nursing students' basic communication and interviewing skills: The development and testing of a rating scale. *Journal of Advanced Nursing, 29*(3), 658-665.

August-Brady, M. M. (2005). The effect of a metacognitive intervention on approach to and self-regulation of learning in baccalaureate nursing students. *Journal of Nursing Education, 44*(7), 297-304.

Ausbel, D., Novak, J., & Hanesian, H. (1978). *Educational psychology: A cognitive view* (2nd ed.). New York: Werbel and Peck.

Bain, K. (2004). *What the best college teachers do.* Cambridge, MA: Harvard University Press.

Barkley, E., Cross, P., & Major, C. H. (2004). *Collaborative learning techniques: A handbook for college faculty.* San Francisco: Jossey-Bass.

Barr, R. B., & Tagg, J. (1995). From teaching to learning: A new paradigm for undergraduate education. *Change, 27*(6), 697-710.

Baxter, P. E., & Boblin, S. L. (2007). The moral development of baccalaureate nursing students: Understanding unethical behavior in classroom and clinical settings. *Journal of Nursing Education, 46*(1), 20-27.

Beckett, A., Gilbertson, S., & Greenwood, S. (2007). Doing the right thing: Nursing students, relational practice, and moral agency. *Journal of Nursing Education, 46*(1), 28-32.

Bekemeier, B. & Butterfield, P. (2005). Unreconciled inconsistencies: A critical review of the concept of social justice in 3 national nursing documents. *Advances in Nursing Science, 28*(2), 152-162.

Benner, P. (2004). Using the Dreyfus model of skill acquisition to describe and interpret skill acquisition and clinical judgment in nursing practice and education. *Bulletin of Science, Technology & Society, 24*, 188-199.

Benner, P., Hooper-Kyriakidis, P., & Stannard, D. (1999). *Clinical wisdom and interventions in critical care: A thinking-in-action approach.* Philadelphia: Saunders.

Benner, P., Sutphen, M., Leonard, V., & Day, L. (2010). *Educating nurses: A call for radical transformation.* San Francisco: Jossey-Bass.

Benner, P. A., Tanner, C. A., & Chesla, C. A. (1996). *Expertise in nursing practice: Caring, clinical judgment, and ethics.* New York: Springer Publishing.

Bennett, K., Sackett, D., Haynes, B., Neufeld, V., Tugwell, P., & Roberts, R. (1987). A controlled trial of teaching critical appraisal of the clinical literature to medical students. *JAMA, 257*(18), 2451-2454.

Berge, Z. (1997). Computer conferencing and the online classroom. *International Journal of Educational Telecommunications, 3*(1), 3-21.

Biggs, J. (1987). *Student approaches to learning and studying.* Melbourne, Victoria: Australian Council for Educational Research, Hawthorn Press.

Bloom, B. J. (1956). *Taxonomy of educational objectives: Cognitive and affective domains.* New York: David McKay.

Boswell, C. (2005). The art of questioning: Improving critical thinking. *Annual Review of Nursing Education, 4*, 291-304.

Boutain, D. M. (2005). Social justice as a framework for professional nursing. *Journal of Nursing Education, 44*(9), 404-408.

Boyer, E. (1990). *Scholarship reconsidered: Priorities of the professoriate.* Princeton, NJ: The Carnegie Foundation for the Advancement of Teaching.

Bransford, J. D., Brown, A. L., & Cocking, R. R. (Eds.). (2004). *How people learn.* Washington, DC: National Academies Press.

Britain, S., & Liber, O. (2004). *A framework for the pedagogical evaluation of virtual learning environments.* Report 41, JISC Technology Applications Programme. Retrieved from http://www.cetis.ac.uk/members/pedagogy/files/4thMeet_frame work/VLEfullReport

Brookfield, S. D., & Preskill, S. (1999). *Discussion as a way of teaching.* San Francisco: Jossey-Bass.

Bruffee, K. (1993). *Collaborative learning.* Baltimore: Johns Hopkins Press.

Bruner, J. (1985). Vygotsky: An historical and conceptual perspective. In J. V. Wertsch (Ed.), *Culture, communication, and cognition: Vygotskian perspectives* (pp. 21-34). London: Cambridge University Press.

Brunt, B. A. (2006). Critical thinking in nursing: An integrative review. *Journal of Continuing Education in Nursing, 36*, 60-67.

Buckingham, M., & Coffman, C. (2004). *First, break all the rules: What the world's greatest managers do differently.* New York: Simon & Schuster.

Byrne, M. M., Weddle, C., Davis, E., & McGinnis, P. (2003). The Byrne guide for inclusionary cultural content. *Journal of Nursing Education, 42*(6), 277-281.

Caelli, K. (1998). Shared understandings: Negotiating the meanings of health via concept mapping. *Nurse Education Today, 18*(4), 317-321.

Camerer, C. F., & Ho, T. H. (2000). *Strategic learning and teaching.* [Monograph.] Pasadena, CA: California Institute of Technology.

Campinha-Bacote, J. (1999). A model and instrument for addressing cultural competence in health care. *Journal of Nursing Education, 38*(5), 203-207.

Candela, L., Dalley, K., & Benzel-Lindley, J. (2006). A case for learning-centered curricula. *Journal of Nursing Education, 45*(2), 59-65.

Cato, M. L., Lasater, K., & Peeples, A. I. (2009). Nursing students' self-assessment of their simulation experiences. *Nursing Education Perspectives, 30*(2), 105-108.

Chant, S., Jenkinson, T., Randle, J., & Russell, G. (2002). Communication skills: Some problems in nursing education and practice. *Journal of Clinical Nursing, 11*(1), 12-21.

Chickering, A. W., & Ehrmann, S. C. (1996). Implementing the seven principles: Technology as lever. *AAHE Bulletin,* October, 3-6. Retrieved from http://www.tltgroup.org/programs/seven.html

Chickering, A. W., & Gamson, Z. F. (1991). *Applying the seven principles of good practice in undergraduate education.* (New Directions for Teaching and Learning, no. 47). San Francisco: Jossey-Bass. Retrieved from http://www.msu.edu/user/coddejos/seven.htm

Clayton, L. H. (2006). An effective, active teaching-learning method. *Nursing Education Perspectives, 27*(4), 197-203.

Collis, B. (1997). *Tele-learning in a digital world: The future of distance learning.* London: International Thomson Computer Press.

Cooke, M., Irby, D. M., O'Brien, B. C., & Shulman, L.S. (2010). Educating physicians: A call for reform of medical school and residency. San Francisco: Jossey-Bass.

Corey, G., Corey, M., & Callanan, P. (2005). An approach to teaching ethics courses in human services and counseling. *Counseling and Values, 49*(3), 193-207.

Cranton, P. (2006). *Understanding and promoting transformative learning: A guide for educators of adults* (2nd ed.). San Francisco: Jossey-Bass.

Daley, B. J., Shaw, C. R., Balistrieri, T., Glasenapp, K., & Piacentine, L. (1999). Concept maps: A strategy to teach and evaluate critical thinking. *Journal of Nursing Education, 38*(1): 42-47.

Davidson, N. (1994). Cooperative and collaborative learning: An integrative perspective. In J. S. Thousand, R. A. Villa & A. I. Nevin (Eds.), *Creativity and collaborative learning: A practical guide to empowering students and teachers* (pp. 13-30). Baltimore: Paul H Brookes.

DeSilets, L. (1986). Self-directed learning in voluntary and mandatory continuing education programs. *Journal of Continuing Education in Nursing, 17*(3), 81-83.

Dillard, N., Sideras, S., Ryan, M., Hodson Carlton, K., Lasater, K., & Siktberg, L. (2009). A collaborative project to apply and evaluate the Clinical Judgment Model through simulation. *Nursing Education Perspectives, 30*(2), 99-104.

Dillon, J. T. (1990). *The practice of questioning.* London: Routledge.

Dolmans, D. H. J. M., Gijselaers, W. H., Moust, J. H. C., De Grave, W. S., Wolfhagen, I. H. A. P., & Van Der Vleuten, C. P. M. (2002). Trends in research on the tutor in problem-based learning: Conclusions and implications for educational practice and research. *Medical Teacher, 24*(2), 173-180.

Dreifuerst, K. T. (2009). The essentials of debriefing in simulation learning: A concept analysis. *Nursing Education Perspectives, 30*(2), 109-114.

Dyck, S. (1986). Self-directed learning for the RN in a baccalaureate program. *Journal of Continuing Education in Nursing, 17*(6), 194-197.

Eagle, C. J., Harasym, P. H., & Mandlin, H. (1992). Effects of tutors with case expertise on problem-based learning issues. *Academic Medicine 67*(7), 465-469.

Elliot, D. D. (1996). Promoting critical thinking in the classroom. *Nurse Educator, 21*(2), 49-52.

Enjelvin, G., & Sutton, A. (2004). 'Let's ask the students for a change.' Investigating student learning approaches to and perceived gains from "VLE-novation". *UCN Working Papers Series, Vol. 1.*

Entwistle, N. (1981). *Styles of learning and teaching: An integrated outline of educational psychology for students, teachers and lecturers.* Chichester, England: John Wiley Chichester.

Ericcson, K. A. (2004). Deliberate practice and the acquisition and maintenance of expert performance in medicine and related domains. *Academic Medicine, 79*(10 Suppl.), S70-S81.

Fanning, R. M., & Gaba, D. M. (2007). The role of debriefing in simulation-based learning. *Simulation in Healthcare, 2*(2), 115-125.

Felder, R. M., & Brent, R. (2001). Effective strategies for cooperative learning. *Journal of Cooperation & Collaboration in College Teaching, 10*(2), 69-75.

Ferrari, E. (2006). Academic education's contribution to the nurse-patient relationship. *Nursing Standard, 21*(10), 35-40.

Fesler-Birch, D. M. (2005). Critical thinking and patient outcomes: A review. *Nursing Outlook, 53*(2), 59-65.

Fineout-Overholt, E., Cox, J., Robbins, B., & Gray, Y. L. (2005). Teaching evidence-based practice. In B. M. Melnyk & E. Fineout-Overholt (Eds.), *Evidence-based practice in nursing and healthcare* (pp. 407-441). Philadelphia: Lippincott, Williams, & Wilkins.

Ford, J. S., & Profetto-McGrath, J. (1994). A model for critical thinking within the context of curriculum as praxis. *Journal of Nursing Education, 33*(8), 341-344.

Foster, C. R. Dahill, L., Golemon, L., & Tolentino, B. W. (2005). *Educating clergy: Teaching practices and pastoral imagination.* San Francisco: Jossey-Bass.

Freeth, D., & Reeves, S. (2004). Learning to work together: Using the presage, process, product (3P) model to highlight decisions and possibilities. *Journal of Interprofessional Care, 18*(1), 43-56.

Furney, S. L., Orsini, A. N., Orsetti, K. E., Stern, D. T., Gruppen, L. D., & Irby, D. M. (2001). Teaching the one-minute preceptor: A randomized controlled trial. *Journal of General Internal Medicine, 16*(9), 620-624.

Gaines, C. (1996). Concept mapping and synthesizers: Instructional strategies for encoding and recalling. *Journal of the New York State Nurses Association, 27*(1), 14-18.

Gerrish, K. (1992). The nurse teacher's role in the practice setting. *Nurse Education Today, 12*(3), 227-232.

Gibbs, G. (1999). Learning how to learn using a virtual learning environment for philosophy. *Journal of Computer Assisted Learning, 15*(3), 221-231.

Gokhale, A. (1995). Collaborative learning enhances critical thinking. *Journal of Technology Education, 7*(1). Retrieved July 5, 2007, from http://scholar.lib.vt.edu/ejournals/JTE/v7n1/gokhale.jte-v7n1.html

Green, M., & Ellis, P. (1997). Impact of evidence-based medicine curriculum based on adult learning theory. *Journal of General Internal Medicine, 12*(12), 742-750.

Greene, M. (1993). Diversity and inclusion: Toward a curriculum for human beings. *Teachers College Record, 95*(2), 211-221.

Gubrud-Howe, P., & Schoessler, M. (2008). From random access opportunity to a clinical education curriculum. *Journal of Nursing Education, 47*(1), 3-4.

Hakkarainen, K., Lipponen, L., & Jaarvela, S. (2002). Epistemology of inquiry and computer-supported collaborative learning. In T. Koschmann, R. Hall, & N. Miyake (Eds.), *CSCL2: Carrying forward the c onversation* (pp. 129-156). Mahwah, NJ: Lawrence Erlbaum Associates.

Hamilton, L., & Gregor, F. (1986). Self-directed learning in a critical care nursing program. *Journal of Continuing Education in Nursing, 17*(3), 94-99.

Hesketh, E. A., Ganall, G., Buckley, E. G., Friedman, M., Goodall, E., Harden, R. M., et al. (2001). A framework for developing excellence as a clinical educator. *Medical Education, 35*(5), 555-564.

Hewitt-Taylor, J. (2001). Self-directed learning: Views of teachers and students. *Journal of Advanced Nursing, 36*(4), 496-504.

Hewson, M. G., & Little, M. L. (1998). Giving feedback in medical education: Verification of recommended techniques. *Journal of General Internal Medicine, 13*(2), 111-116.

Hicks, F. D. (2001). Critical thinking: Toward a nursing science perspective. *Nursing Science Quarterly, 14*(1), 14-21.

Hicks-Moore, S. L., & Pastirik, P. J. (2006). Evaluating critical thinking in clinical concept maps: A pilot study. *International Journal of Nursing Education Scholarship, 3*(1), article 27. Retrieved from http://www.bepress.com/ijnes/vol3/iss1/art27

Hinck, S. M., Webb, P., Sims-Giddens, S., Helton, C., Hope, K. L., Utley, R., et al. (2006). Student learning with concept mapping of care plans in community-based education. *Journal of Professional Nursing, 22*(1), 23-29.

Hoskins, S., & van Hooff, J.C. (2005). Motivation and ability: Which students use online learning and what influence does it have on their achievement? *British Journal of Educational Technology, 36*(2), 177-192.

Hsu, L., & Hsieh, S. (2005). Concept maps as an assessment tool in a nursing course. *Journal of Professional Nursing, 21*(3), 141-149.

Ingersoll, G. (2000). Evidence-based nursing: What it is and what it isn't. *Nursing Outlook, 48*(4), 151-152.

Institute of Medicine. (2003). *Health professions education: A bridge to quality.* Washington, DC: National Academies Press.

Institute of Medicine. (2004). *In the nation's compelling interest: Ensuring diversity in the health care workforce.* Washington, DC: National Academies Press.

Issenberg, S. B., McGaghie, W. C., Petrusa, E. R., Gordon, D. L., & Scalese, R. J. (2005). Features and uses of high-fidelity medical simulations that lead to effective learning: A BEME systematic review. *Medical Teacher, 27*(1), 10-28.

Iwasiw, C. L. (1987). The role of the teacher in self-directed learning. *Nurse Education Today, 7*(5), 222-227.

Jeffries, P. R. (Ed.). (2007). *Simulation in nursing education: From conceptualization to evaluation.* New York: National League for Nursing.

Jelfs, A., & Colbourn, C. (2002). Virtual seminars and their impact on the role of the teaching staff. *Computers and Education, 38*(1-3), 127-136.

Jenkins, M., Browne, T., & Armitage, S. (2001). *Management and implementation of virtual learning environments: A UCISA funded survey.* Retrieved from http://www. ucisa.ac.uk/groups/ssg/surveys.aspx

Jenkins, T. B., Carlson, J. H., & Herrick, C. (1998). Developing self-directed learning modules. *Journal for Nurses in Staff Development, 14*(1), 17-22.

Johnson, D., Johnson, R., & Smith, K. (2007). The state of cooperative learning in postsecondary and professional settings. *Educational Psychology Review, 19*(1), 15-29.

Johnson, T. D., & Ryan, K. E. (2000). A comprehensive approach to the evaluation of college teaching. In K. E. Ryan (Ed.), *Evaluating teaching in higher education: A vision for the future* (New Directions for Teaching and Learning, no. 83, pp. 109-123). San Francisco: Jossey-Bass.

Jonassen, D. H. (2002). Engaging and supporting problem solving in online learning. *Quarterly Review of Distance Education, 3*(1), 1-13.

Jonassen, D. H., & Kwon, H. I. (2001). Communication patterns in computer-mediated vs. face-to-face group problem solving. *Educational Technology: Research and Development, 49*(10), 35-52.

Kaakinen, J., & Arwood, E. (2009). Systematic review of nursing simulation literature for use of learning theory. *International Journal of Nursing Education Scholarship, 6*(1), article 16. Retrieved from http://www.bepress.com/ijnes/vol6/iss1/art16

Kagan, S. (1989/1990). The structural approach to cooperative learning. *Educational Leadership, 47*(4), 12-15.

Kell, C., & Van Deursen, R. (2002). Student learning preferences reflect curricular change. *Medical Teacher, 24*(1), 32-40.

Kinchin, I., & Hay, D. (2005). Using concept maps to optimize the composition of collaborative student groups: A pilot study. *Journal of Advanced Nursing, 51*(2), 182-187.

Kintgen-Andrews, J. (1991). Critical thinking and nursing education: Perplexities and insights. *Journal of Nursing Education, 30*(4), 152-157.

Kluge, M. A., & Glick, L. (2006). Teaching therapeutic communication via camera cues and clues: The video inter-active (VIA) method. *Journal of Nursing Education, 45*(11), 463-468.

Knapper, C. (2001). Broadening our approach to teaching evaluation. In C. Knapper & P. Cranton (Eds.), *Fresh approaches to the evaluation of teaching.* (New Directions for Teaching and Learning, no. 88, pp. 3-9). San Francisco: Jossey-Bass.

Knowles, M. S. (1975). *Self-directed learning: A guide for learners and teachers.* Englewood Cliffs, NJ: Prentice Hall.

Knowles, M. S. (1980). *The modern practice of adult education: From pedagogy to andragogy.* Englewood Cliffs, NJ: Prentice Hall/Cambridge.

Kocaman, G., Dicle, A., & Ugur, A. (2009). A longitudinal analysis of the self-directed learning readiness level of nursing students enrolled in a problem-based curriculum. *Journal of Nursing Education, 48*(5), 286-290.

Kuiper, R. A., & Pesut, D. J. (2004). Cognitive and metacognitive reflective reasoning skills in nursing practice: Self-regulated learning theory. *Journal of Advanced Nursing, 45*(4), 381-391.

Lasater, K. (2007a). High fidelity simulation and the development of clinical judgment: Student experiences. *Journal of Nursing Education, 46*(6), 269-276.

Lasater, K. (2007b). Clinical judgment development: Using simulation to create an assessment rubric. *Journal of Nursing Education, 46*(11), 496-503.

Leigh, G. T. (2008). High-fidelity patient simulation and nursing students' self-efficacy: A review of the literature. *International Journal of Nursing Education Scholarship, 5*(1), article 37. Retrieved from http://www.bepress.com/ijnes/vol5/iss1/art37

Leners, D. W., Roehrs, C., & Piccone, A. V. (2006). Tracking the development of professional values in undergraduate nursing students. *Journal of Nursing Education, 45*(12), 504-511.

Linzer, M., Brown, J., Frazier, L., DeLong, E., & Siegal, W. (1988). Impact of a medical journal club on house-staff reading habits, knowledge, and critical appraisal: A randomized controlled trial. *JAMA, 260*(17), 2537-2541.

Lozano, R. (2001). Needs, practices and recommendations of active learning for today's radiation therapy student. *Radiologic Science and Education, 6*(1), 17-28.

Lunyk-Child, O. I., Crooks, D., Ellis, P. J., Ofosu, C., O'Mara, L., & Rideout, E. (2001). Self-directed learning: Faculty and student perceptions. *Journal of Nursing Education, 40*(3), 116-123.

Lynch, M. (2002). *The online educator: A guide to creating the virtual classroom.* London and New York: Routledge.

Lynch, M. (2005). The promise and practical use of learning objects as an integral strategy for delivery of online learning. In R. C. Sharma, S. Mishra, & S. K. Pulist (Eds.), *Education in the Digital World.* New Delhi, India: Viva Books.

Majumdar, B. (1996). Self-directed learning in the context of a nursing curriculum: Development of a learning plan. *Curationis: South African Journal of Nursing, 19*(2), 43-46.

Mantzoukas, S. (2008). A review of evidence-based practice, nursing research and reflection: Levelling the hierarchy. *Journal of Clinical Nursing, 17*(2), 214-223.

Marton, F., & Saljo, N. (1976). On qualitative differences in learning: 1— Outcome and process. *British Journal of Educational Psychology, 46*(1), 4-11.

Matthews, R. S., Cooper, J. L., Davidson, N., & Hawkes, P. (1995). Building bridges between cooperative and collaborative learning. *Change, 27*(4), 34-37.

McNaught, C., & Lam, P. (2005). Building an evaluation culture and evidence base for e-learning in three Hong Kong universities. *British Journal of Educational Technology, 36*(4), 629-642.

Meleca, B., Schimfhauser, F., Witteman, J., & Sachs, L. (1981). Clinical instruction: A national survey. *Journal of Nursing Education Today, 20*(8), 13-18.

Melnyk, B. M., & Fineout-Overholt, E. (2005). Making the case for evidence-based practice. In B. M. Melnyk, & E. Fineout-Overholt (Eds.), *Evidence-based practice in nursing and healthcare* (pp. 3-24). Philadelphia: Lippincott, Williams, & Wilkins.

Mentkowski, M., Rogers, G., Doherty, A., Loacker, G., Hart, J. R., Rickards, W., et al. (2000). *Learning that lasts: Integrating learning, development, and performance in college and beyond.* San Francisco: Jossey-Bass.

Mezirow, J. (1974). *Priorities for experimentation and development in adult basic education.* New York: Columbia University Press.

Miflin, B. M., Campbell, C. B., & Price, D. A. (2000). A conceptual framework to guide the development of self-directed lifelong learning in problem-based medical curricula. *Medical Education, 34,* 299-306.

Mills J. (1995). Better teaching through provocation. *College Teaching, 46*(1), 21-25.

Mimirinis, M., & Bhattacharya, M. (2007). Design of virtual learning environments for deep learning. *Journal of Interactive Learning Research, 18*(1), 55-64.

Mitchell, P., Stegbauer, C., & Watson, K. (2005, September). Three case studies, three environments. In D. Stevens (Chair), *Redefining professional education: Three case studies.* Symposium conducted at the meeting of the Joint Commission for the Accreditation of Healthcare Agencies, Chicago, IL.

Montgomery, K. (2006). *How doctors think: Clinical judgment and the practice of medicine.* New York: Oxford University Press.

Morin, K. H., & Ashton, K. C. (2004). Research on faculty orientation programs: Guidelines and directions for nurse educators. *Journal of Professional Nursing, 20*(4), 239-250.

Morrison-Beedy, D., Aronowitz, T., Dyne, J., & Mkandawire, L. (2001). Mentoring students and junior faculty in faculty research: A win-win scenario. *Journal of Professional Nursing, 17*(6), 291-296.

Murphy, J. I. (2004). Using focused reflection and articulation to promote clinical reasoning: An evidence-based teaching strategy. *Nursing Education Perspectives, 25*(5), 226-231.

National Council of State Boards of Nursing (NCSBN). (2005, August). [Position paper]. Clinical instruction in prelicensure nursing programs. Retrieved from https://www.ncsbn.org/Final_Clinical_Instr_Pre_Nsg_programs.pdf

National League for Nursing. (2005). *Certified Nurse Educator (CNE) 2005 candidate handbook.* New York: Author.

National League for Nursing. (2006a). [Position statement]. Mentoring of nurse faculty. *Nursing Education Perspectives, 27*(2), 110-113.

Nehring, W. M. (2008). U.S. boards of nursing and the use of high-fidelity patient simulators in nursing education. *Journal of Professional Nursing, 24*(2), 109-117.

Newman, P., & Peile, E. (2002). Valuing learners' experience and supporting further growth: Educational models to help experienced adult learners in medicine. *British Medical Journal, 325*(7357), 200-202.

Nolan, J., & Nolan, M. (1997). Self-directed and student-centered learning in nurse education: 2. *British Journal of Nursing, 6*(2), 103-107.

Noone, L. P., & Swenson, C. (2001). 5 dirty little secrets in higher education. *Educause Review, 36*(6), 20-31.

Norman, G., & Shannon, S. (1998). Effectiveness of instruction in critical appraisal: A critical appraisal. *Canadian Medical Association Journal, 158*(2), 177-181.

Novak, J., & Gowin, D. (1984). *Learning how to learn.* New York: Cambridge University Press.

Oermann, M. H. (1997). Evaluating critical thinking in clinical practice. *Nurse Educator, 22*(5), 25-28.

Oliver, M., & Naidu, S. (1997). Computer supported collaborative reflection in and on action in nursing education. *UltiBase Journal.* Retrieved from http://ultibase.rmit.edu.au/Articles/dec97/oliver1.htm

Pahl, C. (2003). Managing evolution and change in web-based teaching and learning environments. *Computers in Education, 40*, 99-114.

Palmer, P. (1998). *The courage to teach: A guide for reflection and renewal.* San Francisco: Jossey-Bass.

Panitz, T. (2004). Using cooperative learning techniques to establish a student-centered, interactive learning environment. In S. Cassara (Ed.), *Teaching for our times, partnerships and collaborations,* (pp. 22-33). Boston: Bunker Hill Community College.

Paul, R. W., & Heaslip, P. (1995). Critical thinking and intuitive nursing practice. *Journal of Advanced Nursing, 22*(1), 40-47.

Payler, J., Meyer, E., & Humphris, D. (2008). Pedagogy for interprofessional education — what do we know and how can we evaluate it? *Learning in Health and Social Care, 7*(2), 64-78.

Pearson, A., Srivastava, R., Craig, D., Tucker, D., Grinspun, D., Bajnok, I., et al. (2007). Systematic review on embracing cultural diversity for developing and sustaining a healthy work environment in healthcare. *International Journal of Evidence-Based Healthcare, 5*(1), 54-91.

Peters, M. A., & Boylston, M. (2006). Mentoring adjunct faculty: Innovative solutions. *Nursing Educator, 31*(2), 61-64.

Phillips, N., & Duke, M. (2001). The questioning skills of clinical teachers and preceptors: A comparative study. *Journal of Advanced Nursing, 33*(4), 523-532.

Pond, E. F., Bradshaw, M. J., & Turner, S. L. (1991). Teaching strategies for critical thinking. *Nurse Educator, 16*(6), 18-22.

Prociuk. J. L. (1990). Self-directed learning and nursing orientation programs: Are they compatible. *Journal of Continuing Education in Nursing, 21*(6), 252-256.

Profetto-McGrath, J., Smith, K., Day, R., & Yonge, O. (2004). The questioning skills of tutors and students in a context based baccalaureate nursing program. *Nurse Education Today, 24*(5), 363-372.

Rampogus, V. K. (1988). Learning how to learn nursing. *Nurse Education Today, 8*(2), 59-67.

Ramsden, P., & Entwistle, N. J. (1981). Effects of academic departments on students' approaches to studying. *British Journal of Educational Psychology, 51*(3), 368-383.

Rooda, L. A. (1994). Effects of mind mapping on student achievement in a nursing research course. *Nurse Educator, 19*(6), 25-27.

Rudolph, J. W., Simon, R., Dufresne, R., & Raemer, D. B. (2006). There's no such thing as "nonjudgmental" debriefing: A theory and method for debriefing with good judgment. *Simulation in Healthcare, 1*(1), 49-55.

Rudolph, J. W., Simon, R., Raemer, D. B., & Eppich, W. J. (2008). Debriefing as formative assessment: Closing performance gaps in medical education. *Academic Emergency Medicine, 15*(11), 1010-1016.

Russell, A. T., Comello, R., & Wright, D. L. (2007). Teaching strategies promoting active learning in healthcare education. *Journal of Education and Human Development, 1*(1), 1-9.

Russell, T. L. (2001). *The no significant difference phenomenon: A comparative research annotated bibliography on technology for distance education* (5th ed.). Montgomery, AL: International Distance Education Certification Center.

Sackett, D., & Parks, J. (1998). Teaching critical appraisal: No quick fixes. *Canadian Medical Association Journal, 158*(2), 203-204.

Sackett, D. L., Straus, S. E., Richardson, W. S., Rosenberg, W., & Haynes, R. B. (2000). *Evidence-based medicine: How to practice and teach EBM.* London: Churchill Livingstone.

St. Clair, G. (2003). *Beyond degrees: Professional learning for knowledge services.* New York: K.G. Saur.

Schim, S. M., Doorenbos, A. Z., & Borse, N. N. (2005). Cultural competence among Ontario and Michigan healthcare providers. *Journal of Nursing Scholarship, 37*(4), 354-360.

Schmidt, H. C., Van Der Arend, A., Moust, J. H., Kokx, I., & Boon, L. (1993). Influences of tutor's subject-matter expertise on student effort and achievement in problem-based learning. *Academic Medicine, 68*(10), 784-791.

Scholdra, J., & Quiring, J. (1973). The level of questions posed by nursing educators. *Journal of Nursing Education, 12*(3), 15-20.

Schön, D. A. (1987). *Educating the reflective practitioner: Toward a new design for teaching and learning in the professions.* San Francisco: Jossey-Bass.

Schuster, P. (2002). *Concept mapping: A critical thinking approach to care planning.* Philadelphia: F.A. Davis.

Seelig, C. (1991). Affecting residents' literature reading attitudes, behaviors, and knowledge through a journal club intervention. *Journal of General Internal Medicine, 6*(4), 330-334.

Sellappah, S., Hussey, T., Blackmore, A., & McMurray, A. (1998). The use of questioning strategies by clinical teachers. *Journal of Advanced Nursing, 28*(1), 142-148.

Sheppard, S. D., Macatangay, K., Colby, A., & Sullivan, W. M. (2009). *Educating engineers: Designing for the future.* San Francisco: Jossey-Bass.

Shulman, L. (2004). *The wisdom of practice: Essays on teaching, learning, and learning to teach.* San Francisco: Jossey-Bass.

Sigma Theta Tau. (2006). *Mentoring resources.* Retrieved from http://www.nursingsociety. org/Career/CareerMap/Pages/cm_mentoring.aspx

Staib, S. (2003). Teaching and measuring critical thinking. *Journal of Nursing Education, 42*(11), 498-508.

Storey, M. A., Phillips, B., Maczewski, M., & Wang, M. (2002). Evaluating the usability of web-based learning tools. *Educational Technology & Society, 5*(3), 91-100.

Sullivan, W. M., Colby, A., Wegner, J. W., & Bond, L. (2007). *Educating lawyers: Preparation for the profession of the law.* San Francisco: Jossey-Bass.

Sullivan Commission. (2005). Missing persons: Minorities in the health professions: A report of the Sullivan commission on diversity in the health care workforce. Retrieved from http://www.aacn.nche.edu/Media/pdf/SullivanReport.pdf

Tait, H., Entwistle, N. J., & McCune, V. (1998). ASSIST: A reconceptualisation of the approaches to studying inventory. In C. Rust (Ed.), *Improving student learning: Improving students as learners* (pp.262-271). Oxford, UK: Oxford Brookes University, Oxford Centre for Learning Development.

Tanner, C. A. (1998). State of the science: Clinical judgment and evidence-based practice: Conclusions and controversies. *Communicating Nursing Research, 31,* 19-35.

Tanner, C. A. (2001). *Oregon's nursing shortage: A public health crisis in the making.* Portland, OR: Northwest Health Foundation.

Tanner, C. A. (2006). Thinking like a nurse: A research-based model of clinical judgment in nursing. *Journal of Nursing Education, 45*(6), 204-211.

Tomey, A. M. (2003). Learning with cases. *Journal of Continuing Education in Nursing, 34*(1), 34-38.

Udlis, K. A. (2008). Preceptorship in undergraduate nursing education: An integrative review. *Journal of Nursing Education, 47*(1), 20-29.

Vygotsky, L. (1978). *Mind in society: The development of higher psychological processes.* Cambridge, MA: Harvard University Press.

Walsh, C. M., & Seldomridge, L. A. (2006). Critical thinking: Back to square two. *Journal of Nursing Education, 45*(6), 212-219.

Weaver, K., & Morse, J., (2006). Pragmatic utility: Using analytical questions to explore the concept of ethical sensitivity. *Research and Theory for Nursing Practice: An International Journal, 20*(3), 191-214.

Weimer, M. (2002). *Learner-centered teaching: Five key changes to practice.* San Francisco: Jossey-Bass.

Weinberg, L. A., & Stone-Griffith, S. (1992). Alternate methods of teaching: Use of self-learning packets. Journal of Post Anaesthesia Nursing, 7(6), 392-397.

Wheeler, L. A., & Collins, S. K. R. (2003). The influence of concept mapping on critical thinking in baccalaureate nursing students. *Journal of Professional Nursing, 19*(6), 339-346.

Worrell, P. J. (1990). Metacognition: Implications for instruction in nursing education. *Journal of Nursing Education, 29*(4), 170-175.

Glossary

Clinical judgment: Case-based, contextually bound, interpretive reasoning (Tanner, 2006).

Clinical thinking: Clinical judgment and decision-making (Tanner, 2006).

Collaborative learning: Respecting and highlighting individual group members' abilities and contributions while sharing authority and acceptance of responsibility among group members for the group's actions. The process is based upon consensus building through cooperation by group members (Felder & Brent, 2001, Johnson, Johnson & Smith, 2007; Kagan, 1989/1990).

Cooperative learning: Use of a set of processes that help people interact together in order to accomplish a specific goal or develop an end product, which is usually content specific. It is more directive than a collaborative system and more closely controlled by the teacher (Felder & Brent, 2001, Johnson, Johnson & Smith, 2007; Kagan, 1989/1990).

Critical thinking: Praxis; the capability to analyze assumptions, challenge the status quo, recognize limitations in health care, and take action to improve it (Ford & Profetto-McGrath, 1994).

Deep learning: Learning that involves critical analysis and linking of new ideas to already known concepts and principles; which leads to understanding and long-term retention for later use in problem solving within unfamiliar contexts (Biggs, 1987; Entwistle, 1981; Marton & Saljo, 1976). Learning that lasts (Mentkowski et al., 2000).

Faculty development: A process of assisting faculty as they transform their teaching.

Faculty evaluation: A systematic process that considers the faculty member's progress toward an agreed upon set of outcomes across missions in relationship to prespecified criteria or standards.

Learner-centered teaching: "Being learner-centered focuses attention squarely on learning: what the student is learning, how the student is learning, the conditions under which the student is learning, whether the student is retaining and applying the learning, and how current learning positions the student for future learning. The student is still an important part of the equation. In fact, we make the distinction between learner-centered instruction and teacher-centered instruction as a way of indicating that the spotlight has moved from the teacher to student. When instruction is learner-centered, the action focuses on what students (not teachers) are doing." (Weimer, 2002, p. xvi).

Learning-centered teaching: "Learning is an abstraction, and much like content... tends to gravitate toward that which is theoretical and abstract, I want to keep us firmly rooted and fixed on the direct object of our teaching: students. We do not want more and better learning at some abstract level; we need it specifically and concretely for the students we face in class...." (Weimer, 2002, p. xvi).

Metacognition: Thinking about thinking and learning; "Metacognition, a component of executive control, is comprised of both knowledge and skill dimensions. Metacognitive knowledge includes beliefs about one's ability, the demand of a task, and potentially effective learning strategies. Metacognitive skill includes mental acts of self-regulation via planning, predicting, monitoring, regulating, evaluating, and revising strategies. Learning strategies are implemented via metacognitive skills that facilitate intentional learning." (Worrell, 1990, p. 171)

Self-directed learning: "A process in which individuals take the initiative, with or without the help of others, in diagnosing their learning needs, formulating learning goals, identifying human and material resources for learning, choosing and implementing appropriate learning strategies and evaluating learning outcomes." (Knowles, 1975, p. 18)

Strategic learning: Using a combination of deep and surface learning strategies to complete assignments efficiently while attending to the grading criteria in order to perform well (Tait, Entwistle, & McCune, 1998). In the corporate training environment, strategic learning means performance-based learning or "just-in-time" learning (Camerer & Ho, 2000; St. Clair, 2003).

Student-centered teaching: "Being student-centered implies a focus on student needs. It is an orientation that gives rise to the idea of education as a product, with the student as the customer and the role of the faculty as one of serving and satisfying the customer. Faculty resist the student as customer metaphor for some very good reasons. When the product is education, the customer cannot always be right, there is no money-back guarantee, and tuition dollars do not 'buy' the desired grades." (Weimer, 2002, p. xvi).

Surface learning: Tacit acceptance of information and rote memorization of isolated and unlinked facts, leading to superficial retention of material for examinations without understanding or long-term retention of knowledge and information (Biggs, 1987; Entwistle, 1981; Marton & Saljo, 1976).